TRACK YOUR PARENT'S VITAL SIGNS

Vital Signs Record Book

DR. JULIE CRENSHAW

Doctor of Physical Therapy
ABPTS Board Certified Specialist in Geriatrics

Help the Caregiver

ISBN-13: 9781737877622
ISBN-10: 1737877627

Cover design by: 100Covers
Printed in the United States of America

TRACK YOUR PARENT'S VITAL SIGNS

Vital Signs Record Book

How to Use This Book

Welcome to the only vital signs record book you'll ever need!

I designed this book with YOU in mind. In my years working in home health, I have had caregivers express the same concerns over and over when it comes to taking vital signs:

- Am I doing it right?
- Are these numbers good or bad?
- When should I call the doctor?
- WHY is my parent's blood pressure all over the place?!

I answer all of these questions at the front of the book so that you can take your parent's vital signs with confidence AND know what to do with the information once you have it.

Read through these first few pages. I promise they're worth it! Then decide on a consistent routine for tracking vitals every day.

I designed the log to be customizable to your needs. If you take vitals more than once per day, use a new line to track the second and/or third set of vitals. If you only repeat one measure (like blood pressure or blood sugar), use the notes section to log the "PM" measure.

If you are having trouble sorting out blood pressure that seems "all over the place," use the special "Blood Pressure Tracking Chart" in the back of the book for a few weeks and then take it to your cardiologist for analysis.

My Message to You

I know it can feel overwhelming to have to take on this caregiver role. You can easily feel like the weight of the world is on your shoulders and you're fighting to keep your head above water!

I created Help the Caregiver to provide resources, education, and support for caregivers so no one ever has to feel like they're doing this alone again.

Top tips for taking vital signs:

- Take vitals at a **consistent time of day,** preferably **approx 1 hour after taking morning medications.**
- Changes in vitals can be early signs that something is wrong; do not ignore!
- **Use the "troubleshooting guides" in this book** to help identify potential reasons for unusual readings.
- **Communicate with the doctors**; show them this log book so they can quickly recognize trends over time.

If you're not already: make sure you're following me on YouTube.com/@helpthecaregiver and please join my FREE Facebook group:
www.facebook.com/groups/caregiversofaginglovedones

Read on for more detailed instructions and information related to vital signs. Have feedback or questions? Reach out to me at julie@helpthecaregiver.com I'd love to hear from you!

All my best,
Julie

Supply List

You're going to want to make sure you have the right supplies handy in order to feel confident about the vital signs you are taking. Let's go over **my recommendations**. Of course, if your health provider has already given recommendations, follow those guidelines instead.

What's most important is that you are **using the same equipment as much as possible**. Using 3 different blood pressure cuffs and 2 different scales can create problems where there didn't have to be any; even machines can have variation!

If you are interested in the go-to products I recommend, **use your phone's camera to scan the QR code**, or visit www.helpthecaregiver.com/store. Disclaimer: these are affiliate links. There is no extra cost to you for using them, but it puts a little change in my Coffee Fund jar if you do. **I ONLY recommend products that I would use myself or for my loved ones.**

Consider getting the following:

- **Blood pressure cuff**
- **Pulse oximeter** (for checking oxygen and heart rate)
- **Glucometer** (for checking blood sugar)
- **Thermometer**
- **Scale**

Scan with your phone's camera!

Scan this QR code to see all recommended items in one place on my website:

Blood Pressure Cuff

I get asked a lot about my recommendations for blood pressure cuffs. Here's the bottom line: **automatic arm cuffs ARE a great way to take blood pressure!** They are typically very accurate and very reliable.

However, **wrist cuffs are NOT as accurate.** They are a little less expensive, but also less accurate. I highly recommend paying a few extra dollars for a traditional arm cuff. Whatever you choose, just be consistent. Don't use an arm cuff half the time and a wrist cuff the other half. Pick one, and stick with it.

My recommended BP cuff: scan with your phone's camera!

How to use: The cuff I recommend has a picture on it to help guide you in placing the cuff correctly. In general, you want to make sure that the cuff is place on the **upper arm, above the bend in your elbow**, with the **cord that connects the cuff** to the machine **down near the bend of the elbow** (instead of at the "top" near your shoulder). The cord should also be **placed in the "middle" of the elbow/forearm** area instead of off to the side. **Press start** and let the machine take the reading!

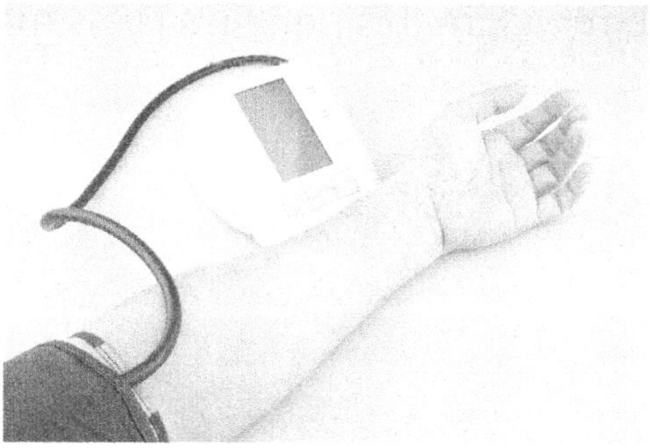

Checking Heart Rate

Heart rate can be checked a few different ways. The only thing I want to emphasize is to be CONSISTENT in how you take heart rate. **Pick a method that you will use for your "official" measure that you will record in this log book, and stick with it.**

You can check it different ways throughout the day to keep an eye on things, but you can cause unnecessary worry if you are checking with multiple different devices.

Options:

1. The **automatic blood pressure cuff** will give you a heart rate reading along with the BP reading
2. The **pulse oximeter** (next page) will give you a heart rate reading along with oxygen reading
3. You might have a **smart watch** of some kind that checks/tracks heart rate. Many of these are accurate, but check it against the BP cuff or oximeter first to make sure before using it as your consistent method.

Pro Tip: If a person has A-FIB, their heart rate will be inconsistent, which confuses automatic devices. It will often show their HR to be MUCH higher than it actually is. The only accurate way to measure this person's HR is manually.

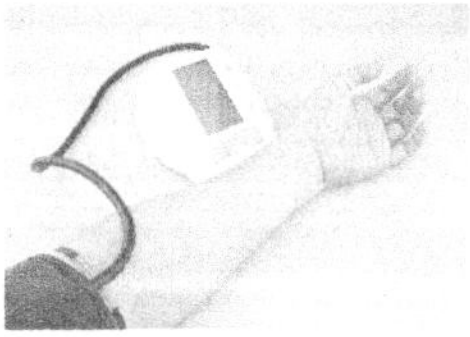

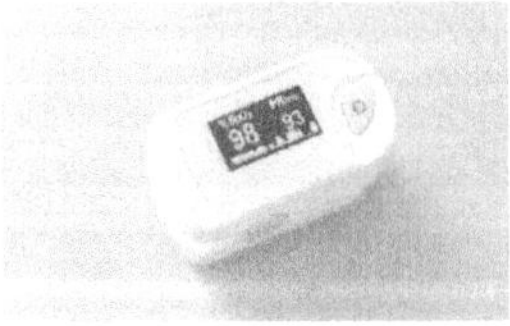

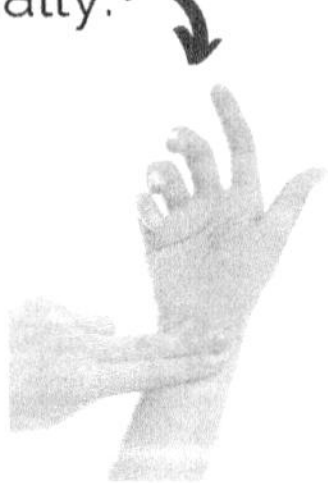

Pulse Oximeter

A pulse oximeter, usually referred to as a "pulse ox," measure the <u>approximate</u> amount of oxygen being carried in a person's blood. This is very important because it shows whether or not a person is getting enough oxygen to function and be healthy.

If their oxygen levels are too low, they could have a lot of difficulty breathing. They could feel exhausted even if they are resting, and if their levels stay too low for long enough, they could start to have bigger health problems.

I highly recommend getting one and keeping it handy if your loved one has trouble breathing or uses oxygen.

My recommended pulse ox: Scan with your phone's camera!

Pro Tips: 1) **The number you see is NOT exact.** We're not going to worry about the difference between 97% and 98%. 2) Although some devices will read oxygen at 100%, this isn't actually possible, medically speaking, so don't worry about getting there. 3) **The most important question is whether or not the person is having trouble breathing**. If you get a crazy low number on the device, but the person insists they feel fine and they're not breathing hard, there is likely a problem with the device itself. 4). **If a person says they are having trouble breathing, even if their oxygen levels are "normal," SEEK IMMEDIATE MEDICAL CARE.** There can be other serious problems that need attention.

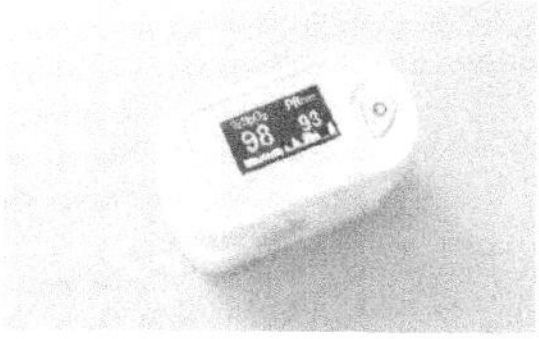

Glucometer

The device that checks **blood sugar** is called a glucometer (it measures glucose levels). For a person with diabetes, it is very important to check blood sugar levels. Having levels that are consistently too high can create damage to nearly every system of the body. Levels that are dangerously low could cause a person to become unresponsive.

It's important to understand that **your body's blood sugar levels are giving you direct feedback about the effects of your diet, exercise, and medication on your body.** Use it as a feedback and investigation tool!

scan with your phone's camera!

My recommended glucometer:

My recommended diabetic diet record book:

How to use: Follow the directions included with the glucometer, but here are the main things to figure out before starting: Make sure you know how to **turn on the device**, how to **use the lancet to pierce the finger**, and **where to put the collection strip** into the device so it can read it.

Pro tip: The lancet has to **pierce deeply enough** to get enough blood. Do it right the first time so you don't have to re-stick! **Warming the finger** first will help get more blood to the area..

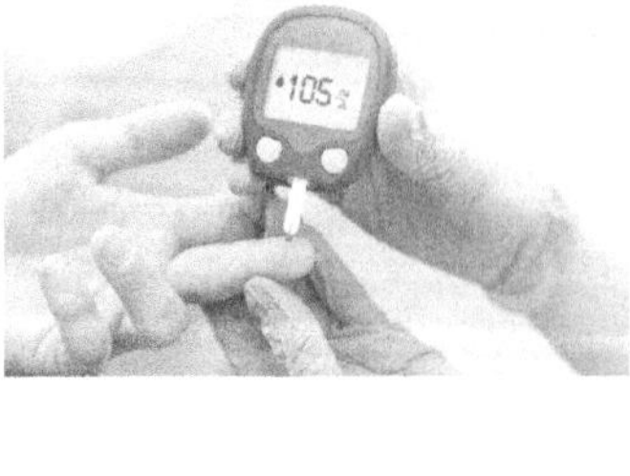

Thermometer

Who knew taking **temperature** could get so confusing with so many thermometers on the market?

I'm going to give you my thoughts about thermometers, but you do what feels right to you, and follow any instructions given by your medical providers.

Traditionally, taking temp orally (by mouth) has always been the gold standard, because other methods were considered less accurate. In my experience working with frail elderly adults, **taking temperature orally isn't ALWAYS the most accurate** because many of my patients are unable to keep the thermometer in the **correct position** (under the tongue) or **fully close their mouths**. This could be due to tremors, stroke, dental problems, inability to follow directions due to advanced dementia, or any number of other reasons.

These problems will effect the accuracy of a reading. Many thermometers today have advanced technology to ensure more accurate readings in alterate locations (forehead, ear, etc). If your loved one can accurately use a traditional thermometer, it will be the least expensive option. If they cannot, an alternate option may be required.

My recommended alternate thermometer:

scan with your phone's camera!

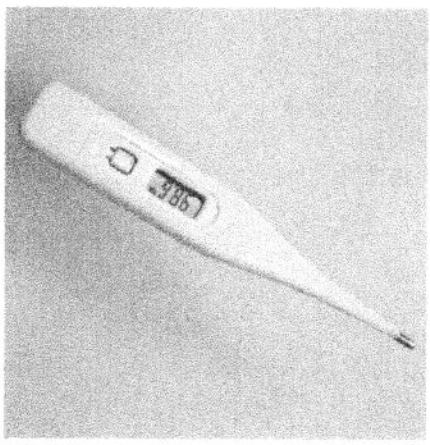

Scale

There are also MANY options on the market for scales that can be used to keep track of weight. As with BP and HR, the most important factor here is consistency. Using different scales at different times can result in too much variation in reading.

Make sure the scale is able to measure a good deal MORE weight than your loved one weighs. If they weigh approx 300 lbs, make sure the scale reads at least 400 lbs. If their weight is too close to the max weight of the scale, it won't be as accurate. **Make sure the batteries are fresh**. Old batteries will start to produce less accurate readings. **Weigh first thing in the morning, after going to the bathroom, with similar weighted clothes on for more accuracy.**

My recommended scale: scan with your phone's camera!

Pro Tip: If your loved one is at a high risk for falls, and standing on a scale is risky, have them walk their walker OVER the top of the scale and hold on to the walker to step onto the scale. Only let go long enough to get the reading, and then grab back onto the walker and carefully step off the scale.

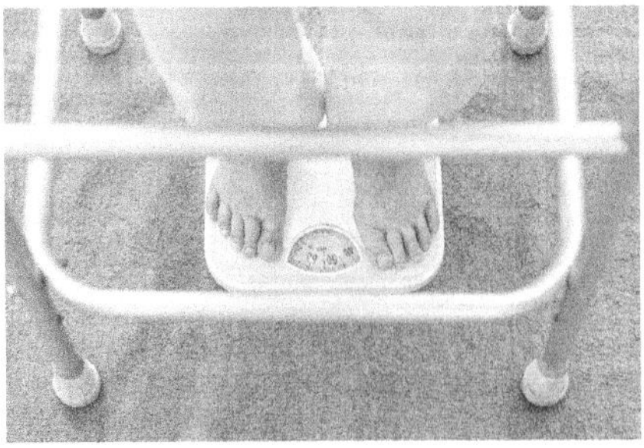

Reference Ranges

It is important to know what is considered NORMAL when you are taking vital signs. After all, what's the point in taking them if you don't know what they mean or what to do with them?

I'm going to provide the STANDARD ranges that are considered normal for most patients. **Your loved one's doctor may want you to use a different range.** There is space below to write alternate instructions from your medical provider.

Not sure who to ask? Ask the doctor who manages the medications for that problem. **That could be the primary doctor or a specialist**. Cardiologist for blood pressure and heart rate. Endocrinologist for blood sugar. Pulmonologist for oxygen levels. Monitoring weight fluctuations could be because of a heart, lung, or kidney problem. Ask the doctor who manages their "water pills" or fluid levels. Still not sure? Ask their primary doctor who should make the call.

	Standard Ranges	MD Preferred
BP (top number)	90-158	____________
BP (bottom number)	60-88	____________
HR	60-100	____________
O2	90-100%	____________
Blood sugar	90-200	____________
Temperature	97.8 - 99.1	____________
Weight	Call for 2+lb gain overnight	____________

See the following page for more information and explanation

When to Call 911

Let's first talk about emergencies that cannot wait, and work our way back from there. **This is NOT a comprehensive list of emergency situations.** This list is related to checking vital signs and abnormal readings from these items.

ALWAYS use your best judgment when deciding to call 911. It doesn't cost anything for the EMT's to come out, evaluate the situation, and give a recommendation. **When in doubt, call!**

If your loved one is having signs or symptoms of a medical problem, checking their vital signs can help you determine what might be going on. You know their medical history and diagnoses, and you can use that information to make a decision about what to do next.

Taking vital signs to report to the 911 dispatcher, and the EMTs, can also help them to give the most appropriate care to your loved one.

If your loved one is experiencing symptoms including dizziness; confusion; headache; chest pain; difficulty breathing, talking, answering questions, or following simple directions (like "raise up both your arms"), they may need emergent medical care.

If they are having **any of these symptoms along with** BP, HR, O2, blood sugar, or weight fluctuations **outside of the ranges** on the previous page **(either too high OR too low)**, you **absolutely need to contact a healthcare professional and/or 911 for help.**

When to Call the MD

I would encourage you to have a conversation with each of your loved one's doctors about WHEN they want you to call them. Many doctors assume that you know when they want to be called, but each doctor is different, so take the time to find out his or her preferences.

Depending on how serious your loved one's condition is, how quickly a change in their status needs to be addressed, and a number of other factors, some doctor's might want to know certain things immediately. Others will simply encourage you to leave a message on the nurse's line if you have a concern.

If you feel overwhelmed by all the doctors, instructions, and logistical information you are trying to keep up with for your loved one, please check out my comprehensive companion log book, "Keeping Up with Your Parent's Doctors All in One." You can get your copy at helpthecaregiver.com/store.

I want to emphasize that in an emergency, you should call 911 or get your loved on to the nearest emergency department or urgent care center. However, there are other times when calling the doctor is the most appropriate choice.

When your loved one's vital signs are outside of the "standard" ranges (or the MD's preferred ranges), **but they are not having any negative symptoms** (headache, dizziness, confusion, etc), we first want to make sure there isn't another explanation for the unusual reading.

When to Call the MD

If this is the first time a reading has been outside of the standard range, or the first time you have seen an unusual number read out for a vital sign, **go to the following "troubleshooting" pages to see if there might be a reasonable explanation** for why your loved one's vital sign is much higher or lower than it normally is.

It could be something as simple as a missed medication or a low battery in a machine, so we want to rule out those things first to avoid unnecessary phone calls, visits, and potentially even tests or medications.

If you've run through the "troubleshooting" pages and have no explanation, it might be that your loved one needs medical attention to get the issue sorted out before it becomes a serious problem.

Call the MD office of the person who manages that condition or medication (go back to the "reference ranges" page for examples). **Let them know about the abnormal reading and ask what they would like you to do next.**

Most of the time, if this is the first time this has happened, they will tell you to keep monitoring their vitals (good thing you have this log book!), but sometimes they may want the patient to come in for a check up.

When you go to the next follow up visit, BRING THIS LOG BOOK WITH YOU so that they can see the many data points you are bringing them, instead of having to rely solely on the vitals they take when you come in.

When to Call the MD

It is very helpful for the doctor to see DAILY vitals for a patient in order to make the best decision about their care and medications.

Blood pressure is one that can be frequently problematic because of "white coat syndrome," which is when a person has a higher BP reading because of anxiety when a healthcare professional takes their BP.

This can make a normal BP seem falsly high, leading to medication prescribed for hypertension unnecessarily, or for a low BP to seem normal, which can delay needed medication for HYPOtension (BP that is so low it can cause dizziness, fatigue, confusion or lethargy). I have seen both of these things happen with my patients in home health.

Please know that you always have the ability to call an MD office and request a visit for a patient to come in and be seen, **even if it is much sooner than their next scheduled appointment.** Doctors make suggestions for when a patient should be seen again based on what they know about that patient and how they are doing at THAT appointment.

They can't possibly know about changes that a patient is having unless someone tells them, and **they WANT you to tell them if something changes so they can help before it becomes serious.**

If you need to: call and schedule an appointment and BRING THIS LOG BOOK to show them what's been going on.

Troubleshooting

When a vital sign reading is out of range, it should not be ignored. **When a vital sign is consistently out of range, it needs to be reported to the doctor** and a follow up appointment may need to be scheduled. However, it is important to look at other potential causes for the reading.

I encourage you to work through these questions (and others that might be related to your situation) to see if you can figure out why a reading might be off.

The purpose of this is two-fold. First, you don't want to call the doctor or 911 just to realize later that the batteries in your machine were dying, and that's the reason you had a crazy reading.

The second is to see if there were any lifestyle factors (what the patient did or didn't eat, forgetting to take a medication, etc) that caused a less than ideal vital sign reading, but ALSO was avoidable.

When you can play detective and figure these things out, you can learn more about the cause and effect of these actions so that you can set yourself/the patient up for better success next time.

It's all about learning how to manage the situation in front of you. It might be finding a better snack for the end of the day, or it might be that the doctor needs to prescribe a new or different medication.

Going through this process with help you know which is right.

Blood Pressure

If BP is too high, ask the following questions:

- Has the person missed any of their blood pressure medications?
- Are they feeling very stressed or anxious? (Either of these can drive BP up).
- Have they eaten any foods with a lot of salt in the last 24 hours?
- Have they smoked in the last 30 minutes?

If the answer to all of these is "no," take BP again, either in the other arm, or in the same arm after waiting 5 minutes. A top number >160 needs to be brought down under 160 asap. A top number >180 is an emergency whether the person has symptoms or not. Report to the nearest emergency room.

If BP is too low, ask the following questions:

- If they take a medicine for low BP, have they missed a dose?
- If they take medicine for high BP, did they accidentally take more than one dose?
- Have they started or changed a new BP medication in the last week or two?
- Are they possibly dehydrated? Exhausted from spending the day out of the house?
- Are any of their other vital signs out of range? (There could be several things going on at once here.)

Low BP will often come with symptoms of light-headedness or fatigue. If the answer to all the above questions is "no," I would still encourage you to give your loved one a healthy snack and some water. Reassess in 30 minutes to an hour.

Heart Rate

If **heart rate is too high**, ask the following questions:

- Is the person feeling anxious or stressed?
- Has the person just finished exercising or done more activity than usual today? (Sometimes the stress of being so fatigued can temporarily increase heart rate)
- Could they be dehydrated? (Dehydration can often show in vital signs as low BP combined with high HR.)
- Are they having trouble breathing? (This can cause physical or emotional stress that can increase HR.)
- Do they have a-fib? (The only accurate way to check HR when a person has a-fib is to check it manually.)

If the answer to all of these questions is "no," and the person isn't having any symptoms, continue to monitor, and report to primary doctor or cardiologist if it persists. It could be an indication of a new problem that needs to be checked.

If **heart rate is too low**, ask the following questions:

- Could the person have accidentally taken too much high blood pressure medication?
- Did they forget to take a medication that brings their HR up?
- Have they taken too much pain medicine?
- Are they dehydrated? (Yes, dehydration can cause high OR low blood pressure)
- Is their blood sugar also very low?

Low heart rate can be the result of too much medication or blood sugar "bottoming out." Monitor closely and call 911 if it doesn't come up after eating a healthy snack and drink.

Oxygen

If a person is "on oxygen," they will **not likely have oxygen levels that are too high.** UNLESS their pulmonologist (lung doctor) has told you that their oxygen needs to stay under a certain number.

For some people with lung disease, their body is not capable of breathing "normally" anymore, and they must maintain their oxygen levels closer to 88-90%. This only applies to your loved one if they have been specifically told to keep levels there by their doctor. WRITE THIS DOWN ON THE REFERENCE RANGE SECTION OF THIS BOOK.

If this is true for your loved one, ask the MD what to do if their O2 levels are "too high." Do they want you to turn down how many liters of oxygen they are on until they are in the optimal range? This sort of information can be logged in your "Keeping Up with Your Parent's Doctors All in One" log book.

Normal, healthy lungs will not produce low oxygen numbers, no matter how out of breath a person is. If your loved one has a low oxygen reading, they are **having trouble breathing and they are NOT "on oxygen," they need to report to the emergency room.**

If they are "on oxygen," their numbers are low, and they are having only a little more trouble breathing than usual, use your judgement to consider calling their doctor first to see if they want you to turn the oxygen up, come in to be seen, or to report to the emergency room.

Severe trouble breathing is an emergency. Call 911!

Blood Sugar

Blood sugar is something that can be so frustrating and overwhelming to get under control. Most people don't check blood sugar unless they have a diagnosis of diabetes. I will focus here on Type 2 diabetes and will only cover the points I most commonly go over with my older patients:

Tips and Facts:

- "Sugar free" products are NOT healthy and do very little to help maintain healthy blood sugar levels. Eat more vegetables and drink water.
- Eating high sugar foods at night (like ice cream) is probably CAUSING your blood sugar to bottom out while you sleep. Stop doing it.
- If you "have" to eat something you know will increase your blood sugar, eat it at lunch and get up and move around after. Don't eat the carbs and sugar at night before bed!
- Pain can cause an increase in blood sugar. Monitor blood sugar levels more closely after surgery or injury.
- Going for a short walk (even up and down the hall a few times!) will help bring insulin levels down after a meal.
- The best thing you can do is to keep track of what you eat, how much you move, and what your blood sugar readings are so you can best understand how YOUR body is effected by specific foods and types of movement.

In order to learn more about your body and how to manage your blood sugar, I recommend this diabetic journal:

Make sure you have clear instructions from your doctor about what he or she wants you to do, medication and diet wise, **when your blood sugar levels are too high or too low.**

Temperature

If **temperature is too high**, ask the following questions:

- How hot is it in the room? If it's the middle of summer in the south and there's no air conditioning, and everyone is sweating, that may be effecting temperature.
- Is the person sitting next to a space heater? Those can create so much heat in the immediate space that a reading can be falsely high.
- If you are taking temperature by mouth, did the person just drink scalding hot coffee?

If **temperature is too low**, ask the following questions:

- (If taking by mouth): is the person able to put and keep the thermometer under their tongue with their mouth fully closed? If not, another method of taking temperature is more appropriate.
- (If taking with a temp "gun": is this a low quality product that is taking inaccurate readings on everyone? (Check temp on other people to see what a typical reading is.)
- For all methods: are the batteries running low? (Low batteries will frequently lead to inaccurate readings.)

There is no point in taking temperature if you aren't going to get an accurate reading, and MANY products on the market take poor quality readings. Also, if a person cannot keep a thermometer under their tongue with their mouth fully closed, an oral thermometer will not be able to give an accurate reading.

Make sure to read the instructions on "touchless" temp guns to know how closely to hold it to the skin for good readings.

Weight

The reason you are likely checking weight daily is to keep an eye on fluid levels. If your loved one is on lasix (a "water pill"), then it is extremely important to check weight every single day.

The reason for this is because taking on extra fluid weight is one of the first signs of a heart failure problem getting worse. If it can be caught in time, it can frequently be corrected by taking extra medication (ONLY if you are directed to do that by your doctor!).

If not caught, or ignored, it can quickly lead to a lengthy stay in the hospital.

The body cannot create several pounds of fat overnight, but it can definitely retain several pounds of fluid! That's why the standard instructions are to call the doctor if you experience a 2 pound weight gain overnight.

Your doctor may want that to be a slightly different number, so **ASK the doctor 1) how much weight gain is a concerning amount? 2) What do I do if that much weight is gained?** (Call the MD, take an extra pill, report to emergency room, etc).

Write any instructions about how much weight gain is "too much" on the reference range page of this book. Put any further instructions in your "Keeping Up with Your Parent's Doctors All in One" log book.

Remember: you have to weigh EVERY DAY to know when the gain happened. TAKE THIS LOG BOOK TO YOUR MD VISIT.

Identifying Patterns

The last thing I want to cover here is about recognizing when something is headed in the wrong direction, before it becomes a serious problem or emergency situation.

One of the great advantages of taking daily vital signs is the ability to know what is "normal" for your loved one, and what isn't. For example, my blood pressure tends to be around 96/62 the majority of the time. This is normal for me. If my blood pressure were to read 134/78, this would be a huge increase for me, and something I would be concerned about!

BUT 134/78 is what my husband's blood pressure tends to be most of the time, so that reading wouldn't be concerning at all for him. For him, a reading of 96/62 would be serious cause for concern! It would indicate a large drop in pressure that we would want to have checked out.

If you are taking daily vitals and notice that something was very consistent for a long time (in this example, blood pressure), and then **you notice that over a period of a few weeks, or over a month, that the number has been trending upward or downward by a change of 10 or more, this is something to bring up to the doctor.**

Ex. Blood pressure in the 130's, then 140's, then 150's...

If left alone, it's likely that the number will continue in that direction until it gets into an extreme range that could lead to an emergency. **If you notice this, CALL THE DOCTOR! Explain the changes and ask for a visit**. BRING THIS LOG BOOK to show them what you are seeing.

Confusing BP?!

Blood pressure makes sense when it's consistently high or low. They make medication for that!

We also just went over what to do when you see blood pressure trending upward or downward by a lot, and to call the doctor if you see that happening. They make medication for that!

BUT, what if blood pressure seems all over the place? It's too high one time, and then too low the next, and then normal for a few days, and then there's another randomly high reading??

It's enough to make you feel crazy! I have had this happen to MANY of my patients working in home health, and I have come up with a chart for them that has helped to solve many cases of "Wild" blood pressure readings that seemed to make no sense.

If this is something your loved one is dealing with, head to the back of this log book for further information, instructions, and a special blood pressure tracking chart that will help you and your doctor get to the bottom of what is going on.

Once you have BP under control, go back to logging it as usual in the pages that follow. There are multiple pages of the special BP tracking chart in the back in case you need to go back through that process at a later date.

Vital Signs

DATE	BP	HR	O2	BLOOD SUGAR	TEMP	WEIGHT	NOTES
4/1	**132/74**	**68**	**98**	**124**	**98.1**	**172.3**	**Sample**

Vital Signs

DATE	BP	HR	O2	BLOOD SUGAR	TEMP	WEIGHT	NOTES

Vital Signs

DATE	BP	HR	O2	BLOOD SUGAR	TEMP	WEIGHT	NOTES

Vital Signs

DATE	BP	HR	O2	BLOOD SUGAR	TEMP	WEIGHT	NOTES

Vital Signs

DATE	BP	HR	O2	BLOOD SUGAR	TEMP	WEIGHT	NOTES

Vital Signs

DATE	BP	HR	O2	BLOOD SUGAR	TEMP	WEIGHT	NOTES

Vital Signs

DATE	BP	HR	O2	BLOOD SUGAR	TEMP	WEIGHT	NOTES

Vital Signs

DATE	BP	HR	O2	BLOOD SUGAR	TEMP	WEIGHT	NOTES

Vital Signs

DATE	BP	HR	O2	BLOOD SUGAR	TEMP	WEIGHT	NOTES

Vital Signs

DATE	BP	HR	O2	BLOOD SUGAR	TEMP	WEIGHT	NOTES

Vital Signs

DATE	BP	HR	O2	BLOOD SUGAR	TEMP	WEIGHT	NOTES

Vital Signs

DATE	BP	HR	O2	BLOOD SUGAR	TEMP	WEIGHT	NOTES

Vital Signs

DATE	BP	HR	O2	BLOOD SUGAR	TEMP	WEIGHT	NOTES

Vital Signs

DATE	BP	HR	O2	BLOOD SUGAR	TEMP	WEIGHT	NOTES

Vital Signs

DATE	BP	HR	O2	BLOOD SUGAR	TEMP	WEIGHT	NOTES

Vital Signs

DATE	BP	HR	O2	BLOOD SUGAR	TEMP	WEIGHT	NOTES

Vital Signs

DATE	BP	HR	O_2	BLOOD SUGAR	TEMP	WEIGHT	NOTES

Vital Signs

DATE	BP	HR	O2	BLOOD SUGAR	TEMP	WEIGHT	NOTES

Vital Signs

DATE	BP	HR	O2	BLOOD SUGAR	TEMP	WEIGHT	NOTES

Vital Signs

DATE	BP	HR	O2	BLOOD SUGAR	TEMP	WEIGHT	NOTES

Vital Signs

DATE	BP	HR	O2	BLOOD SUGAR	TEMP	WEIGHT	NOTES

Vital Signs

DATE	BP	HR	O2	BLOOD SUGAR	TEMP	WEIGHT	NOTES

Vital Signs

DATE	BP	HR	O2	BLOOD SUGAR	TEMP	WEIGHT	NOTES

Vital Signs

DATE	BP	HR	O2	BLOOD SUGAR	TEMP	WEIGHT	NOTES

Vital Signs

DATE	BP	HR	O2	BLOOD SUGAR	TEMP	WEIGHT	NOTES

Vital Signs

DATE	BP	HR	O2	BLOOD SUGAR	TEMP	WEIGHT	NOTES

Vital Signs

DATE	BP	HR	O2	BLOOD SUGAR	TEMP	WEIGHT	NOTES

Vital Signs

DATE	BP	HR	O2	BLOOD SUGAR	TEMP	WEIGHT	NOTES

Vital Signs

DATE	BP	HR	O2	BLOOD SUGAR	TEMP	WEIGHT	NOTES

Vital Signs

DATE	BP	HR	O2	BLOOD SUGAR	TEMP	WEIGHT	NOTES

Vital Signs

DATE	BP	HR	O2	BLOOD SUGAR	TEMP	WEIGHT	NOTES

Vital Signs

DATE	BP	HR	O2	BLOOD SUGAR	TEMP	WEIGHT	NOTES

Vital Signs

DATE	BP	HR	O2	BLOOD SUGAR	TEMP	WEIGHT	NOTES

Vital Signs

DATE	BP	HR	O2	BLOOD SUGAR	TEMP	WEIGHT	NOTES

Vital Signs

DATE	BP	HR	O2	BLOOD SUGAR	TEMP	WEIGHT	NOTES

Vital Signs

DATE	BP	HR	O2	BLOOD SUGAR	TEMP	WEIGHT	NOTES

Vital Signs

DATE	BP	HR	O2	BLOOD SUGAR	TEMP	WEIGHT	NOTES

Vital Signs

DATE	BP	HR	O2	BLOOD SUGAR	TEMP	WEIGHT	NOTES

Vital Signs

DATE	BP	HR	O2	BLOOD SUGAR	TEMP	WEIGHT	NOTES

Vital Signs

DATE	BP	HR	O2	BLOOD SUGAR	TEMP	WEIGHT	NOTES

Vital Signs

DATE	BP	HR	O2	BLOOD SUGAR	TEMP	WEIGHT	NOTES

Vital Signs

DATE	BP	HR	O2	BLOOD SUGAR	TEMP	WEIGHT	NOTES

Vital Signs

DATE	BP	HR	O2	BLOOD SUGAR	TEMP	WEIGHT	NOTES

Vital Signs

DATE	BP	HR	O2	BLOOD SUGAR	TEMP	WEIGHT	NOTES

Vital Signs

DATE	BP	HR	O2	BLOOD SUGAR	TEMP	WEIGHT	NOTES

Vital Signs

DATE	BP	HR	O2	BLOOD SUGAR	TEMP	WEIGHT	NOTES

Vital Signs

DATE	BP	HR	O_2	BLOOD SUGAR	TEMP	WEIGHT	NOTES

Vital Signs

DATE	BP	HR	O2	BLOOD SUGAR	TEMP	WEIGHT	NOTES

Vital Signs

DATE	BP	HR	O2	BLOOD SUGAR	TEMP	WEIGHT	NOTES

Vital Signs

DATE	BP	HR	O2	BLOOD SUGAR	TEMP	WEIGHT	NOTES

Vital Signs

DATE	BP	HR	O2	BLOOD SUGAR	TEMP	WEIGHT	NOTES

Vital Signs

DATE	BP	HR	O2	BLOOD SUGAR	TEMP	WEIGHT	NOTES

Vital Signs

DATE	BP	HR	O2	BLOOD SUGAR	TEMP	WEIGHT	NOTES

Vital Signs

DATE	BP	HR	O2	BLOOD SUGAR	TEMP	WEIGHT	NOTES

Sorting Out BP

If your blood pressure readings seem "all over the place," it's something that you likely want to sort out and get under control. Not only can it make you feel awful to have large swings in your blood pressure, it's dangerous and can cause overwhelm and anxiety.

With my patients, there is usually either **1) a timing issue of WHEN their BP medications are being taken** and/or **2) a dosage issue of how much medication is being prescribed or taken at once.**

For this process, you will fill out this chart for at least 14 days, but usually no more than 4 weeks. Make an appointment with your doctor to show him or her this chart and come up with a plan of action. After your BP is under control, go back to taking it as usual and logging in the main charting section of this book.

When you wake up in the morning, your blood pressure is the highest it will be all day. Between the hormone changes that happen during our daily wake/sleep cycle and the length of time since you've had a BP pill, it will be highest when you first wake up.

TAKE YOUR BP FIRST THING WHEN YOU WAKE UP so you know how high it's getting overnight. Also, write down the time that you have woken up and are taking this blood pressure reading. Having big changes in your wake up time can have a big effect on your BP because it changes WHEN you take your first medications and how closely together you take all your other medications after that.

Sorting Out BP

Taking medication at 9a, 12p, 5p, and 9p one day and then taking them at 12p, 3:30p, 6:30p, and 9:30p the next because you slept until noon WILL have a big effect on your BP!

Next: **your BP medications will take full effect somewhere around an hour after you take them.** This means that about an hour after taking your pill, you will know the maximum effect that your medications are having on your BP.

For this process, you are going to take your blood pressure a LOT for 2-4 weeks. It might feel annoying and tedious, but if you want quick, helpful answers to what is going on, just do it! (This is my bossy-but-helpful side coming out. You're welcome.)

So **AFTER YOU TAKE YOUR WAKE UP BP, TAKE YOUR MORNING BP PILLS.** Then, **TAKE YOUR BLOOD PRESSURE AGAIN AN HOUR LATER**. Does your blood pressure get down to "normal," or is it still sky high an hour later? If it's still too high, that pill did not have a strong enough effect.

Did your BP bottom out an hour later? Maybe that pill is too strong, or maybe you're taking more than one pill that effects your BP, and those pills need to be taken at different times from each other.

TAKE YOUR BLOOD PRESSURE AGAIN RIGHT BEFORE YOU TAKE YOUR NEXT DOSE OF BP MEDICATION. This way you will know how high your BP is getting between doses.

Sorting Out BP

Maybe your BP is through the roof before your next dose, which might indicate that you need to take that dose sooner or that the pill you took needed to be stronger to last longer.

Maybe your BP is still in a normal range, so taking that next dose so soon is actually bringing your BP too low, and you might need to change your schedule to take that dose later in the day.

You're going to go through this process for as many times a day as you take BP medication. I've put room for up to 4 doses of BP medication/day. It is extremely uncommon to take BP medication more often than that.

Only take it once/day? Go through the morning process, and then check BP again half way through the day and at the end of the day around bed time.

Take it 2x/day? Take your BP a minimum of 3 times every day: morning, half way through the day, and again at the end of the day. Take BP 1 hour after each dose of medication.

As I've mentioned several times in this log book CONSISTENCY is the key. Not only with the devices you use to take vitals, but with the TIMES you are taking your medications.

Writing down the TIMES you are taking these readings is also extremely important information for your doctor to help you.

SHOW YOUR DOCTOR THIS LOG SHEET!

Blood Pressure

	WAKE UP & 1ST PILL	1 HR LATER	2ND PILL	1 HR LATER	3ND PILL	1 HR LATER	4TH PILL	1 HR LATER
Date	All night without meds	Effect of 1st pill	Highest BP gets b/t pills	Effect of 2nd pill	Highest BP gets b/t pills	Effect of 3rd pill	Highes t BP gets b/t pills	Effect of 4th pill
Ex.	**158/86 8:30a**	**126/78** 9:30a	**146/84 12:30p**	**122/76** 1:30p	**144/82 5:30p**	**124/74** 6:30p	**140/76 8:30p**	**120/72** 9:30p

1. Take BP first thing after you wake up
2. Take BP with each dose of medicine
3. Take BP 1 hour after each dose of medicine
4. Take BP a minimum of 3x/day - when you first wake up, half way through your waking hours, and before bed.
5. Be CONSISTENT with times for taking BP and medications
6. After 2-4 weeks, take this chart to your cardiologist for analysis

Blood Pressure

WAKE UP & 1ST PILL	1 HR LATER	2ND PILL	1 HR LATER	3ND PILL	1 HR LATER	4TH PILL	1 HR LATER

Date	All night without meds	Effect of 1st pill	Highest BP gets b/t pills	Effect of 2nd pill	Highest BP gets b/t pills	Effect of 3rd pill	Highest BP gets b/t pills	Effect of 4th pill

Blood Pressure

	WAKE UP & 1ST PILL	1 HR LATER	2ND PILL	1 HR LATER	3ND PILL	1 HR LATER	4TH PILL	1 HR LATER
Date	All night without meds	Effect of 1st pill	Highest BP gets b/t pills	Effect of 2nd pill	Highest BP gets b/t pills	Effect of 3rd pill	Highes t BP gets b/t pills	Effect of 4th pill

Blood Pressure

	WAKE UP & 1ST PILL	1 HR LATER	2ND PILL	1 HR LATER	3ND PILL	1 HR LATER	4TH PILL	1 HR LATER
Date	All night without meds	Effect of 1st pill	Highest BP gets b/t pills	Effect of 2nd pill	Highest BP gets b/t pills	Effect of 3rd pill	Highest BP gets b/t pills	Effect of 4th pill

Blood Pressure

	WAKE UP & 1ST PILL	1 HR LATER	2ND PILL	1 HR LATER	3ND PILL	1 HR LATER	4TH PILL	1 HR LATER
Date	All night without meds	Effect of 1st pill	Highest BP gets b/t pills	Effect of 2nd pill	Highest BP gets b/t pills	Effect of 3rd pill	Highes t BP gets b/t pills	Effect of 4th pill

Blood Pressure

WAKE UP & 1ST PILL	1 HR LATER	2ND PILL	1 HR LATER	3ND PILL	1 HR LATER	4TH PILL	1 HR LATER	
Date	All night without meds	Effect of 1st pill	Highest BP gets b/t pills	Effect of 2nd pill	Highest BP gets b/t pills	Effect of 3rd pill	Highest BP gets b/t pills	Effect of 4th pill

Blood Pressure

	WAKE UP & 1ST PILL	1 HR LATER	2ND PILL	1 HR LATER	3ND PILL	1 HR LATER	4TH PILL	1 HR LATER
Date	All night without meds	Effect of 1st pill	Highest BP gets b/t pills	Effect of 2nd pill	Highest BP gets b/t pills	Effect of 3rd pill	Highest BP gets b/t pills	Effect of 4th pill

Blood Pressure

	WAKE UP & 1ST PILL	1 HR LATER	2ND PILL	1 HR LATER	3ND PILL	1 HR LATER	4TH PILL	1 HR LATER
Date	All night without meds	Effect of 1st pill	Highest BP gets b/t pills	Effect of 2nd pill	Highest BP gets b/t pills	Effect of 3rd pill	Highes t BP gets b/t pills	Effect of 4th pill

Blood Pressure

	WAKE UP & 1ST PILL	1 HR LATER	2ND PILL	1 HR LATER	3ND PILL	1 HR LATER	4TH PILL	1 HR LATER
Date	All night without meds	Effect of 1st pill	Highest BP gets b/t pills	Effect of 2nd pill	Highest BP gets b/t pills	Effect of 3rd pill	Highes t BP gets b/t pills	Effect of 4th pill

Blood Pressure

	WAKE UP & 1ST PILL	1 HR LATER	2ND PILL	1 HR LATER	3ND PILL	1 HR LATER	4TH PILL	1 HR LATER
Date	All night without meds	Effect of 1st pill	Highest BP gets b/t pills	Effect of 2nd pill	Highest BP gets b/t pills	Effect of 3rd pill	Highest BP gets b/t pills	Effect of 4th pill

Blood Pressure

	WAKE UP & 1ST PILL	1 HR LATER	2ND PILL	1 HR LATER	3ND PILL	1 HR LATER	4TH PILL	1 HR LATER
Date	All night without meds	Effect of 1st pill	Highest BP gets b/t pills	Effect of 2nd pill	Highest BP gets b/t pills	Effect of 3rd pill	Highes t BP gets b/t pills	Effect of 4th pill

Blood Pressure

	WAKE UP & 1ST PILL	1 HR LATER	2ND PILL	1 HR LATER	3ND PILL	1 HR LATER	4TH PILL	1 HR LATER
Date	All night without meds	Effect of 1st pill	Highest BP gets b/t pills	Effect of 2nd pill	Highest BP gets b/t pills	Effect of 3rd pill	Highest BP gets b/t pills	Effect of 4th pill

ABOUT

DR. JULIE CRENSHAW

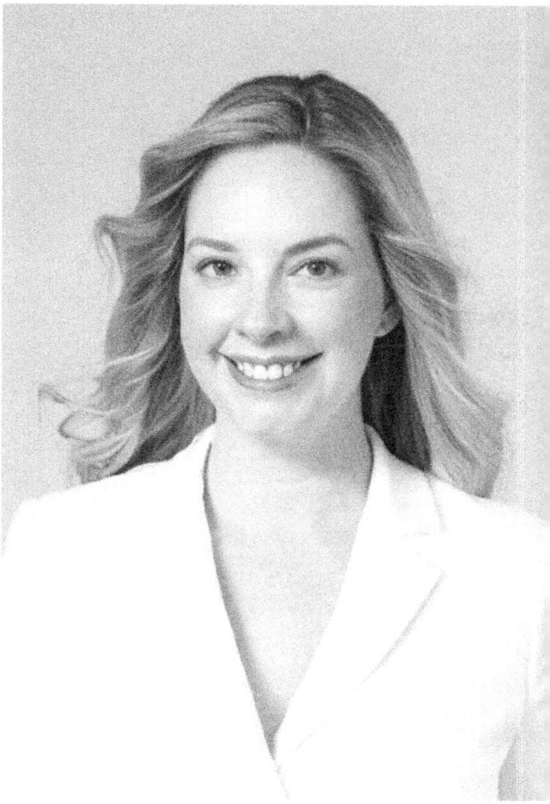

Julie started college as a music performance major playing the french horn, but ultimately pursued becoming a physical therapist to be able to give hands-on care to others. It didn't take long after graduating PT school for Julie to realize the passion she felt for working with the aging population.

It was her many years of working in home health that inspired her to found Help the Caregiver in order to create change for caregivers who she saw doing so much with so little help.

Julie was born and raised in Georgia, where she currently lives with her husband and 3 children.

She loves spending quality time with her family any way that will put her near water, whether it's by the beach, lake, pool, or hiking to a beautiful waterfall.

Books in this Series

Learn to Care for Aging Parents

The "Learn to Care for Aging Parents" series is designed for caregivers in order to empower them with knowledge and decrease overwhelm related to caring for aging loved ones.

This set of 3 books makes the perfect resource for new and long-term caregivers alike, helping to give structure and organization to caregiving needs.

Use the vital signs and MD communication log books to track important measures and keep medical information well organized. Practical tips, checklists, and troubleshooting guides available in the "Bringing a Parent Home from the Hospital" resource book give important information that can be referred to again and again.

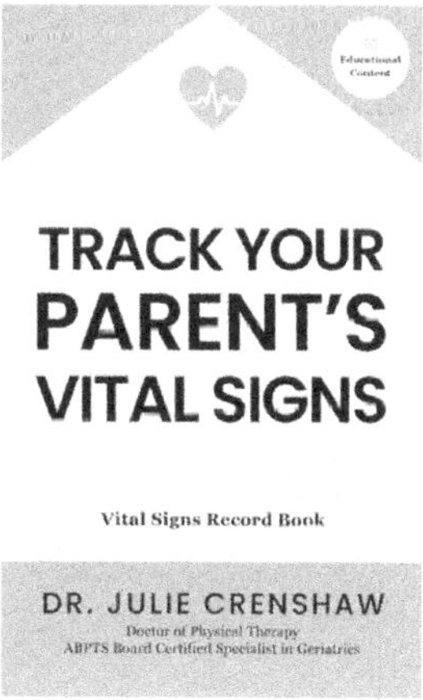

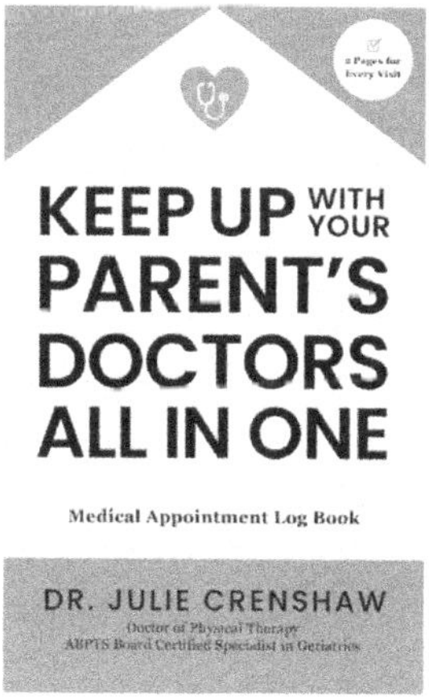

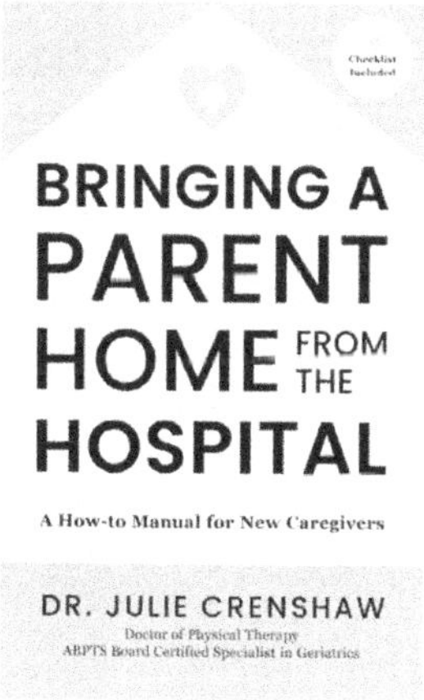

Made in the USA
Monee, IL
04 November 2026

67386528R00056